Alkaline Dinner Cookbook

A collection of delicious recipes for your Alkaline dinner

Isaac Vinson

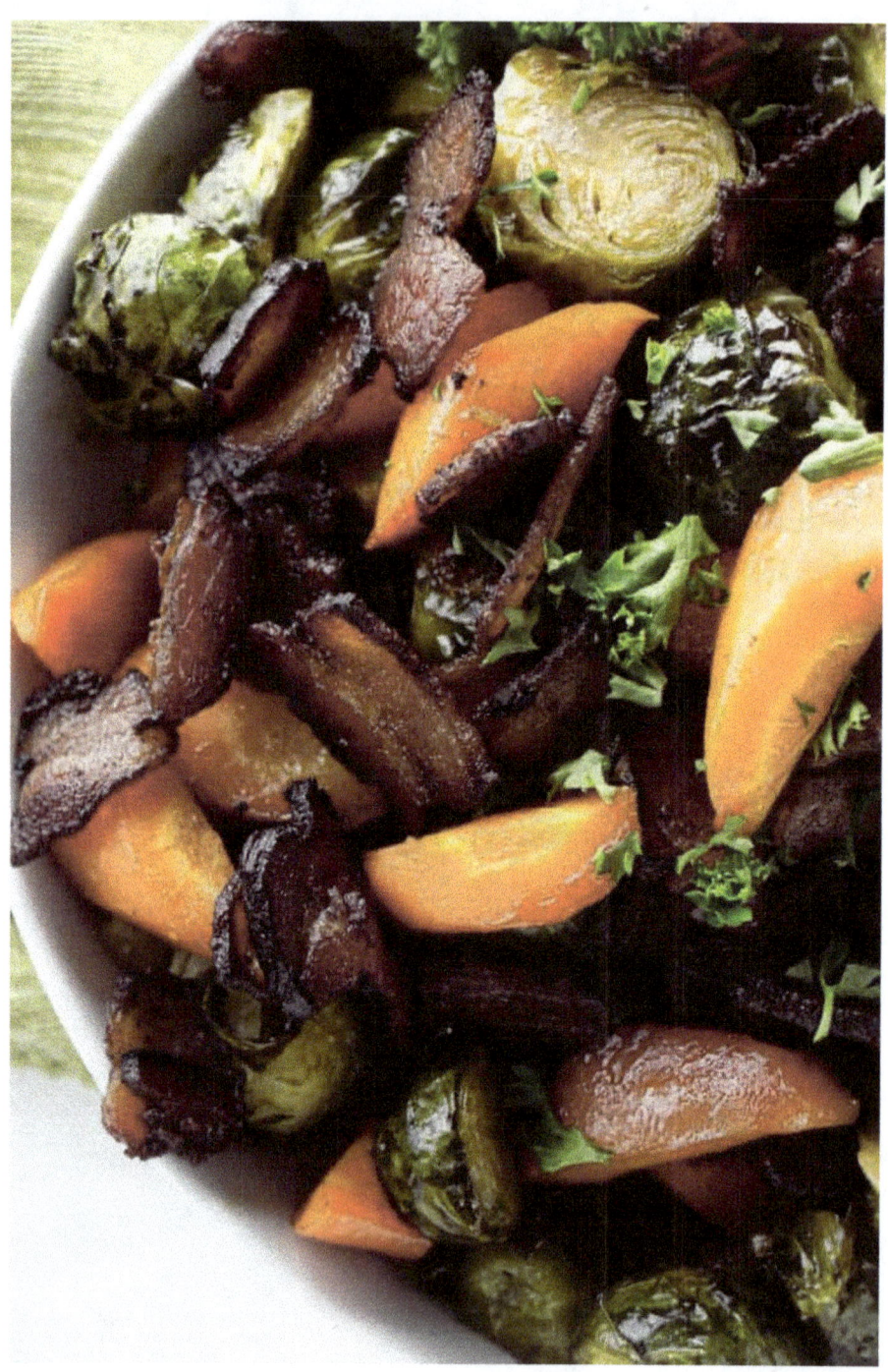

© copyright 2021 – all rights reserved.

the content contained within this book may not be reproduced, duplicated or transmitted without direct written permission from the author or the publisher.

under no circumstances will any blame or legal responsibility be held against the publisher, or author, for any damages, reparation, or monetary loss due to the information contained within this book. either directly or indirectly.

legal notice:

this book is copyright protected. this book is only for personal use. you cannot amend, distribute, sell, use, quote or paraphrase any part, or the content within this book, without the consent of the author or publisher.

disclaimer notice:

please note the information contained within this document is for educational and entertainment purposes only. all effort has been executed to present accurate, up to date, and reliable, complete information. no warranties of any kind are declared or implied. readers acknowledge that the author is not engaging in the rendering of legal, financial, medical or professional advice. the content within this book has been derived from various sources. please consult a licensed professional before attempting any techniques outlined in this book.

by reading this document, the reader agrees that under no circumstances is the author responsible for any losses, direct or indirect, which are incurred as a result of the use of information contained within this document, including, but not limited to, — errors, omissions, or inaccuracies.

Table of Contents

- BRUSSELS SPROUTS & CARROTS 5
- CAJUN SEASONED ZUCCHINI 7
- FRIED CABBAGE 9
- TOFU CURRY 12
- WHOLE CAULIFLOWER WITH GRAVY 14
- MISTO QUENTE 17
- GARLIC BREAD 20
- BRUSCHETTA 22
- CREAM BUNS WITH STRAWBERRIES 24
- BLUEBERRY BUNS 26
- CAULIFLOWER POTATO MASH 29
- FRENCH TOAST IN STICKS 31
- MUFFINS SANDWICH 33
- BACON BBQ 35
- STUFFED FRENCH TOAST 37
- SCALLION SANDWICH 40
- LEAN LAMB AND TURKEY MEATBALLS WITH YOGURT 42
- AIR FRIED SECTION AND TOMATO 45
- CHEESY SALMON FILLETS 47
- SALMON WITH ASPARAGUS 49
- SHRIMP IN GARLIC BUTTER 51
- COBB SALAD 53
- SEARED TUNA STEAK 55
- BEEF CHILI 57
- GREEK BROCCOLI SALAD 60
- CHEESY CAULIFLOWER GRATIN 62
- STRAWBERRY SPINACH SALAD 64
- CAULIFLOWER MAC & CHEESE 66
- EASY EGG SALAD 69
- BAKED CHICKEN LEGS 71
- CREAMED SPINACH 73

STUFFED MUSHROOMS	75
VEGETABLE SOUP	78
PORK CHOP DIANE	80
AUTUMN PORK CHOPS WITH RED CABBAGE AND APPLES	82
CHIPOTLE CHILI PORK CHOPS	84
ORANGE-MARINATED PORK TENDERLOIN	86
HOMESTYLE HERB MEATBALLS	88
LIME-PARSLEY LAMB CUTLETS	90
MEDITERRANEAN STEAK SANDWICHES	92
ROASTED BEEF WITH PEPPERCORN SAUCE	94
COFFEE-AND-HERB-MARINATED STEAK	97
TRADITIONAL BEEF STROGANOFF	99
CHICKEN AND ROASTED VEGETABLE WRAPS	101
SPICY CHICKEN CACCIATORE	103

Brussels Sprouts & Carrots

Preparation Time: 10 minutes.
Cooking Time: 5 minutes.
Servings: 6

Ingredients :

- 1 ½ lb. Brussels sprouts, trimmed and cut in half

- 4 carrots peel and cut in thick slices

- 1 tsp. olive oil

- ½ cup filtered alkaline water

- 1 tbsp. dried parsley

- ¼ tsp. garlic, chopped

- ¼ tsp. pepper

- ¼ tsp. sea salt

Directions:

1. Add all Ingredients into the instant pot and stir well.

2. Seal pot with lid and cook on manual high pressure for 2 minutes.

3. When finished, release pressure using the quick-release method than open the lid.

4. Stir well and serve.

Nutrition:

Calories: 73

Fat: 1. 2 g.

Carbohydrates: 14. 5 g.

Sugar: 4. 5 g.

Protein: 4. 2 g.

Cajun Seasoned Zucchini

Preparation Time: 8 minutes.

Cooking Time: 2 minutes.

Servings: 2

Ingredients :

- 4 zucchinis, sliced

- 1 tsp. garlic powder

- 1 tsp. paprika

- 2 tbsp. Cajun seasoning

- ½ cup filtered alkaline water

- 1 tbsp. olive oil

Directions:

1. Add all Ingredients into the instant pot and stir well.

2. Seal pot with lid and cook on low pressure for 1 minute.

3. When finished, release pressure using the quick-release method than open the lid.

4. Stir well and serve.

Nutrition:

Calories: 130

Fat: 7. 9 g.

Carbohydrates: 14. 7 g.

Sugar: 7. 2 g.

Protein: 5. 3 g.

Cholesterol: 0 mg.

Fried Cabbage

Preparation Time: 10
Cooking Time: 3 minutes.
Servings: 6

Ingredients :

- 1 head cabbage, chopped
- ½ tsp. chili powder
- ½ onion, diced
- ½ tsp. paprika
- 1 onion, chopped
- 1 cup filtered alkaline water
- 2 tbsp. olive oil
- ½ tsp. sea salt

Directions:

1. Add olive oil into the instant pot and set the pot on sauté mode.

2. Add the onion in olive oil and sauté until softened.

3. Add remaining Ingredients and stir to combine.

4. Seal pot with lid and cook on high pressure for 3 minutes.

5. When finished, release pressure using the quick-release method than open the lid.

6. Stir well and serve.

Nutrition:
Calories: 75

Fat: 4. 9 g.

Carbohydrates: 8 g.

Sugar: 4. 2 g.

Protein: 1. 7 g.

Cholesterol: 0 mg.

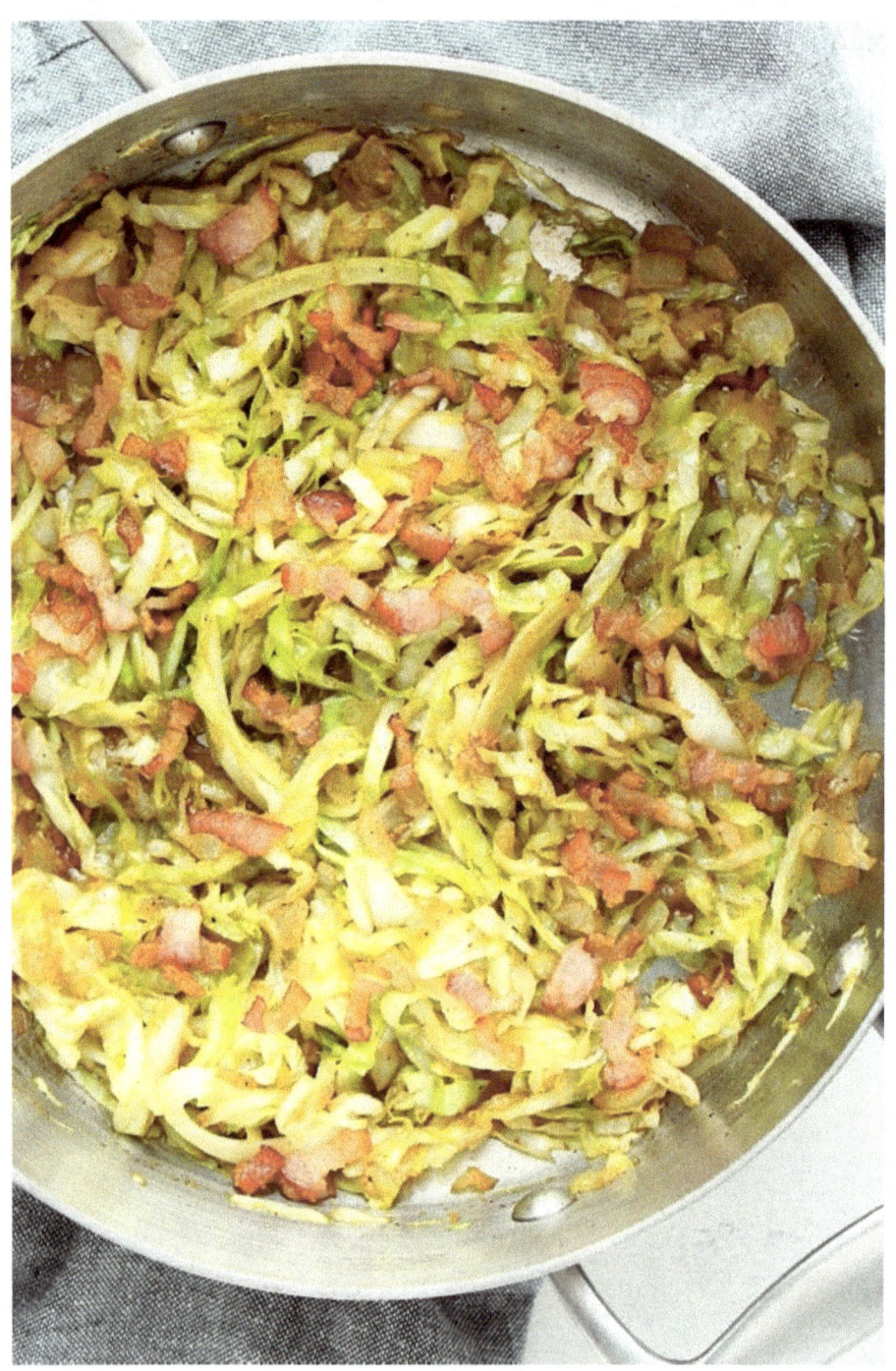

Whole Cauliflower With Gravy

Preparation Time: 10 minutes.
Cooking Time: 15 minutes.

Servings: 5

Ingredients :

- 1 large cauliflower head, cut bottom leaves

For marinade:

- 1 tsp. paprika ½ tbsp. olive oil

- Tbsp. fresh parsley, chopped

- 1 tbsp. fresh thyme

- 3 garlic cloves

- Pepper

- Salt

For gravy:

- ½ tbsp. lime juice

- ½ tsp. thyme

- 1 ½ cups filtered alkaline water

- 2 garlic cloves

- 1 tsp. olive oil

- 1 onion, diced

Directions:

1. In a small bowl, mix together all marinade Ingredients.

2. Rub marinade evenly all over cauliflower head.

3. For the gravy: add oil in an instant pot and set the pot on sauté mode.

4. Add garlic and onion in olive oil and sauté until onion is softened.

5. Add water, lemon juice, and thyme and stir well.

6. Place trivet in the instant pot. Place cauliflower head on a trivet.

7. Seal pot with lid and cook on manual high pressure for 3 minutes.

8. When finished, allow releasing pressure naturally for 5 minutes then release using a quick-release method.

9. Transfer cauliflower head to an oven-safe dish and broil for 3–4 minutes.

10. Puree the instant pot gravy using an immersion hand blender until smooth.

11. Set instant pot on sauté mode and cook the gravy for 3–4 minutes.

12. Serve cauliflower with gravy.

Nutrition:
Calories: 79

Fat: 2. 7 g.

Carbohydrates: 12. 7 g.

Sugar: 5. 1 g.

Protein: 3. 9 g.

Cholesterol: 0 mg.

Misto Quente

Preparation Time: 5 minutes
Cooking Time: 10 minutes
Servings: 4

Ingredients :

- 4 slices of bread without shell

- 4 slices of turkey breast

- 4 slices of cheese

- 2 tbsp. cream cheese

- 2 spoons of butter

Directions:

1. Preheat the air fryer. Set the timer of 5 minutes and the temperature to 200C.

2. Pass the butter on one side of the slice of bread, and on the other side of the slice, the cream cheese.

3. Mount the sandwiches placing two slices of turkey breast and two slices cheese between the breads, with the cream cheese inside and the side with butter.

4. Place the sandwiches in the basket of the air fryer. Set the timer of the air fryer for 5 minutes and press the power button.

Nutrition:

Calories: 340

Fat: 15g

Carbohydrates: 32g

Protein: 15g

Sugar: 0g

Cholesterol: 0mg

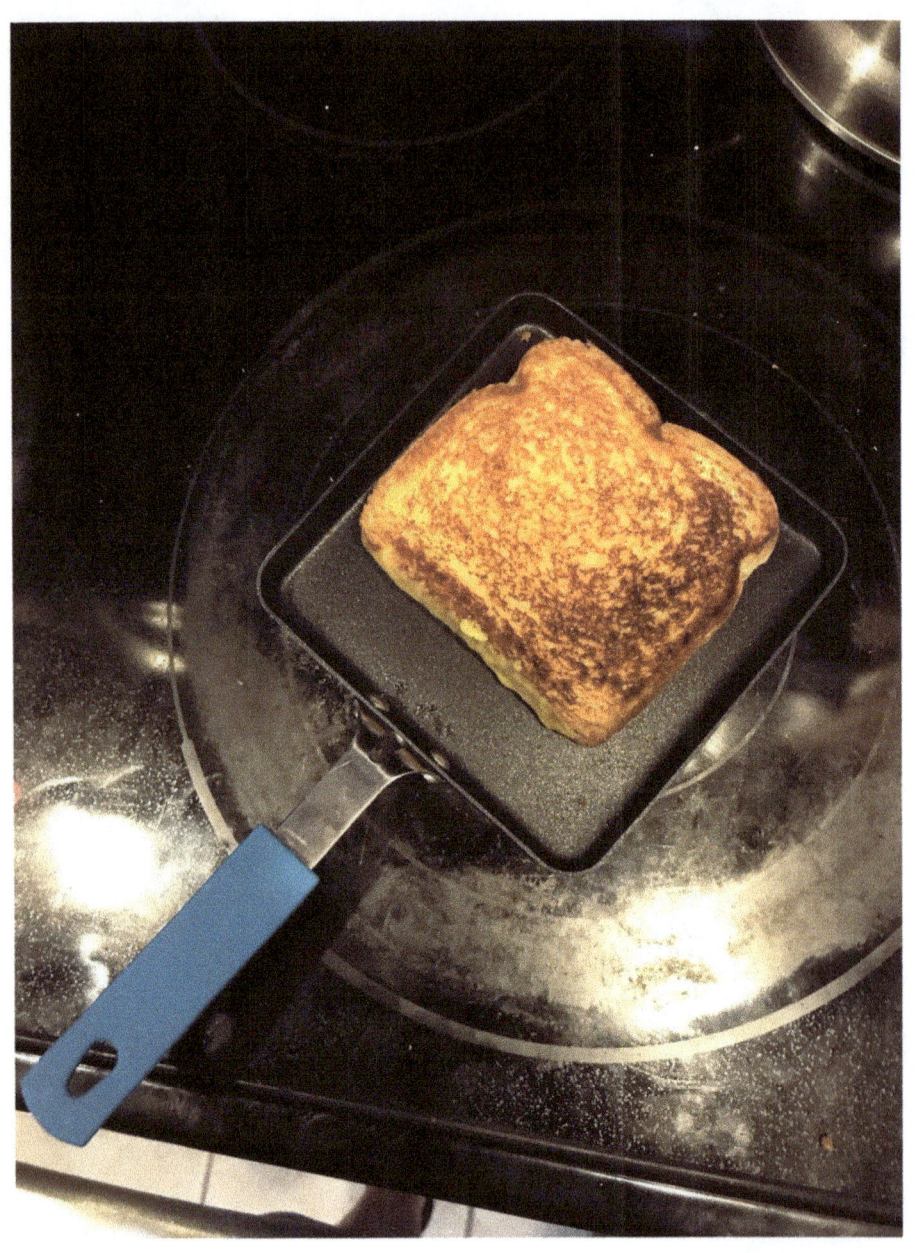

Garlic Bread

Preparation Time: 10 minutes
Cooking Time: 15 minutes
Servings: 4-5

Ingredients :

- 2 stale French rolls

- 4 tbsp. crushed or crumpled garlic

- 1 cup of mayonnaise

- Powdered grated Parmesan

- 1 tbsp. olive oil

Directions:

1. Preheat the air fryer. Set the time of 5 minutes and the temperature to 200oC.

2. Mix mayonnaise with garlic and set aside.

3. Cut the baguettes into slices, but without separating them completely.

4. Fill the cavities of equals. Brush with olive oil and sprinkle with grated cheese.

5. Place in the basket of the air fryer. Set the timer to 10 minutes, adjust the temperature to 180oC and press the power button.

Nutrition:

Calories: 340

Fat: 15g

Carbohydrates: 32g

Protein: 15g

Sugar: 0g

Cholesterol: 0mg

Bruschetta

Preparation Time: 5 minutes
Cooking Time: 10 minutes
Servings: 2

Ingredients :

- 4 slices of Italian bread

- 1 cup chopped tomato tea

- 1 cup grated mozzarella tea

- Olive oil

- Oregano, salt, and pepper

- 4 fresh basil leaves

Directions:

1. Preheat the air fryer. Set the timer of 5 minutes and the temperature to 200oC.

2. Sprinkle the slices of Italian bread with olive oil. Divide the chopped tomatoes and mozzarella between the slices. Season with salt, pepper, and oregano.

3. Put oil in the filling. Place a basil leaf on top of each slice.

4. Put the bruschetta in the basket of the air fryer being careful not to spill the filling. Set the timer of 5 minutes, set the temperature to 180C, and press the power button.

5. Transfer the bruschetta to a plate and serve.

Nutrition:

Calories: 434

Fat: 14g

Carbohydrates: 63g

Protein: 11g

Sugar: 8g

Cholesterol: 0mg

Cream Buns With Strawberries

Preparation Time: 10 minutes

Cooking Time: 12 minutes

Servings: 6

Ingredients :

• 240g all-purpose flour

• 50g granulated sugar

• 8g baking powder

• 1g of salt

• 85g chopped cold butter

• 84g chopped fresh strawberries

• 120 ml whipping cream

• 2 large eggs

• 10 ml vanilla extract

• 5 ml of water

Directions:

1. Sift flour, sugar, baking powder and salt in a large bowl. Put the butter with the flour with the use of a blender or your hands until the mixture resembles thick crumbs.

2. Mix the strawberries in the flour mixture. Set aside for the mixture to stand. Beat the whipping cream, 1 egg and the vanilla extract in a separate bowl.

3. Put the cream mixture in the flour mixture until they are homogeneous, and then spread the mixture to a thickness of 38 mm.

4. Use a round cookie cutter to cut the buns. Spread the buns with a combination of egg and water. Set aside

5. Preheat the air fryer, set it to 180C.

6. Place baking paper in the preheated inner basket.

7. Place the buns on top of the baking paper and cook for 12 minutes at 180C, until golden brown.

Nutrition:
Calories: 150Fat: 14g

Carbohydrates: 3g

Protein: 11g

Sugar: 8g

Cholesterol: 0mg

Blueberry Buns

Preparation Time: 10 minutes
Cooking Time: 12 minutes
Servings: 6

Ingredients :

- 240g all-purpose flour

- 50g granulated sugar

- 8g baking powder

- 2g of salt

- 85g chopped cold butter

- 85g of fresh blueberries

- 3g grated fresh ginger

- 113 ml whipping cream

- 2 large eggs

- 4 ml vanilla extract

- 5 ml of water

Directions:

1. Put sugar, flour, baking powder and salt in a large bowl.

2. Put the butter with the flour using a blender or your hands until the mixture resembles thick crumbs.

3. Mix the blueberries and ginger in the flour mixture and set aside

4. Mix the whipping cream, 1 egg and the vanilla extract in a different container.

5. Put the cream mixture with the flour mixture until combined.

6. Shape the dough until it reaches a thickness of approximately 38 mm and cut it into eighths.

7. Spread the buns with a combination of egg and water. Set aside Preheat the air fryer set it to 180C.

8. Place baking paper in the preheated inner basket and place the buns on top of the paper. Cook for 12 minutes at 180C, until golden brown

Nutrition:
Calories: 105
Fat: 1. 64g
Carbohydrates: 20.09g
Protein: 2. 43g

Sugar: 2.1g
Cholesterol: 0mg

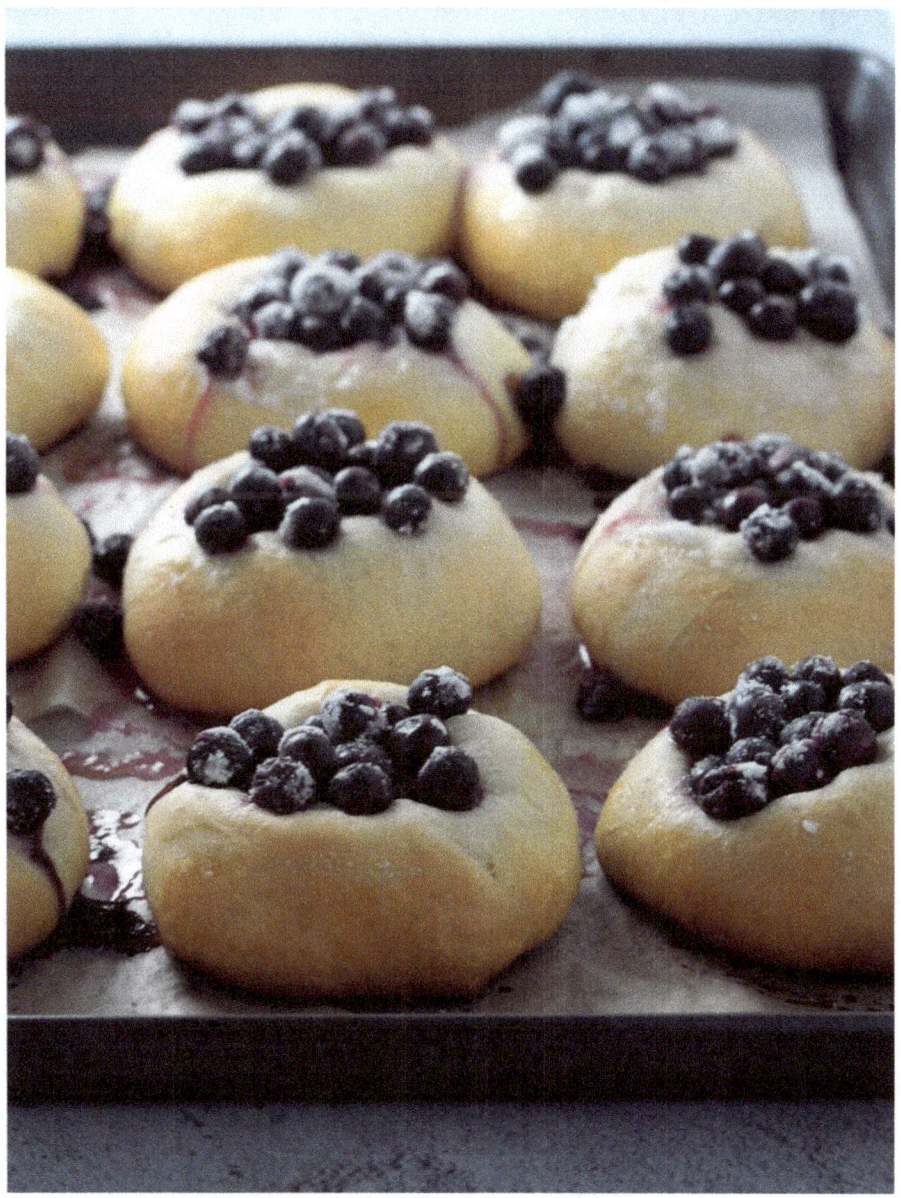

Cauliflower Potato Mash

Preparation Time: 30 minutes
 Servings: 4
Cooking Time: 5 minutes

Ingredients :

- 2 cups potatoes, peeled and cubed

- 2 tbsp. butter

- ¼ cup milk

- 10 oz. cauliflower florets

- ¾ tsp. salt

Directions:

1. Add water to the saucepan and bring to boil.

2. Reduce heat and simmer for 10 minutes.

3. Drain vegetables well. Transfer vegetables, butter, milk, and salt in a blender and blend until smooth.

4. Serve and enjoy.

Nutrition:

Calories 128

Fat 6. 2 g,

Sugar 3. 3 g,

Protein 3. 2 g,

Cholesterol 17 mg

French Toast In Sticks

Preparation Time: 5 minutes
Cooking Time: 10 minutes
Servings: 4

Ingredients :

- 4 slices of white bread, 38 mm thick, preferably hard

- 2 eggs

- 60 ml of milk

- 15 ml maple sauce

- 2 ml vanilla extract

- Nonstick Spray Oil

- 38g of sugar

- 3ground cinnamon

- Maple syrup, to serve

- Sugar to sprinkle

Directions:

1. Cut each slice of bread into thirds making 12 pieces. Place sideways

2. Beat the eggs, milk, maple syrup and vanilla.

3. Preheat the air fryer, set it to 175C.

4. Dip the sliced bread in the egg mixture and place it in the preheated air fryer. Sprinkle French toast generously with oil spray.

5. Cook French toast for 10 minutes at 175C. Turn the toast halfway through cooking.

6. Mix the sugar and cinnamon in a bowl.

7. Cover the French toast with the sugar and cinnamon mixture when you have finished cooking.

8. Serve with Maple syrup and sprinkle with powdered sugar

Nutrition:

Calories 128

Fat 6. 2 g,

Carbohydrates 16. 3 g,

Sugar 3. 3 g,

Protein 3. 2 g,

Cholesterol 17 mg

Muffins Sandwich

Preparation Time: 2 minutes
Cooking Time: 10 minutes
Servings: 1

Ingredients :
- Nonstick Spray Oil

- 1 slice of white cheddar cheese

- 1 slice of Canadian bacon

- 1 English muffin, divided

- 15 ml hot water

- 1 large egg

- Salt and pepper to taste

Directions:

1. Spray the inside of an 85g mold with oil spray and place it in the air fryer.

2. Preheat the air fryer, set it to 160C.

3. Add the Canadian cheese and bacon in the preheated air fryer.

4. Pour the hot water and the egg into the hot pan and season with salt and pepper.

5. Select Bread, set to 10 minutes.

6. Take out the English muffins after 7 minutes, leaving the egg for the full time.

7. Build your sandwich by placing the cooked egg on top of the English muffing and serve

Nutrition:
Calories 400

Fat 26g,

Carbohydrates 26g,

Sugar 15 g,

Protein 3 g,

Cholesterol 155 mg

Bacon BBQ

Preparation Time: 2 minutes
Cooking Time: 8 minutes
Servings: 2

Ingredients :

- 13g dark brown sugar

- 5g chili powder

- 1g ground cumin

- 1g cayenne pepper

- 4 slices of bacon, cut in half

Directions:

1. Mix seasonings until well combined.

2. Dip the bacon in the dressing until it is completely covered. Leave aside.

3. Preheat the air fryer, set it to 160C.

4. Place the bacon in the preheated air fryer

5. Select Bacon and press Start/Pause.

Nutrition:

Calories: 1124

Fat: 72g

Carbohydrates: 59g

Protein: 49g

Sugar: 11g

Cholesterol: 77mg

Stuffed French Toast

Preparation Time: 4 minutes
Cooking Time: 10 minutes
Servings: 1

Ingredients :

- 1 slice of brioche bread,

- 64 mm thick, preferably rancid

- 113g cream cheese

- 2 eggs

- 15 ml of milk

- 30 ml whipping cream

- 38g of sugar

- 3g cinnamon

- 2 ml vanilla extract

- Nonstick Spray Oil

- Pistachios chopped to cover

- Maple syrup, to serve

Directions:

1. Preheat the air fryer, set it to 175C.

2. Cut a slit in the middle of the muffin.

3. Fill the inside of the slit with cream cheese. Leave aside.

4. Mix the eggs, milk, whipping cream, sugar, cinnamon, and vanilla extract.

5. Moisten the stuffed French toast in the egg mixture for 10 seconds on each side.

6. Sprinkle each side of French toast with oil spray.

7. Place the French toast in the preheated air fryer and cook for 10 minutes at 175C

8. Stir the French toast carefully with a spatula when you finish cooking.

9. Serve topped with chopped pistachios and acrid syrup.

Nutrition:

Calories: 159

Fat: 7. 5g

Carbohydrates: 25. 2g

Protein: 14g

Sugar: 0g

Cholesterol: 90mg

Scallion Sandwich

Preparation Time: 10 minutes
Cooking Time: 10 minutes
Servings: 1

Ingredients :

- 2 slices wheat bread

- 2 teaspoons butter, low fat

- 2 scallions, sliced thinly

- 1 tablespoon of parmesan cheese, grated

- 3/4 cup of cheddar cheese, reduced fat, grated

Directions:

1. Preheat the Air fryer to 356 degrees.

2. Spread butter on a slice of bread. Place inside the cooking basket with the butter side facing down.

3. Place cheese and scallions on top. Spread the rest of the butter on the other slice of bread Put it on top of the sandwich and sprinkle with parmesan cheese.

4. Cook for 10 minutes.

Nutrition:

Calorie: 154

Carbohydrate: 9g

Fat: 2. 5g

Protein: 8. 6g

Fiber: 2. 4g

Lean Lamb And Turkey Meatballs With Yogurt

Preparation Time: 10 minutes
Servings: 4
Cooking Time: 8 minutes

Ingredients :

- 1 egg white

- 4 ounces ground lean turkey

- 1 pound of ground lean lamb

- 1 teaspoon each of cayenne pepper, ground coriander, red chili pastes, salt, and ground cumin

- 2 garlic cloves, minced

- 1 1/2 tablespoons parsley, chopped

- 1 tablespoon mint, chopped

- 1/4 cup of olive oil

For the yogurt

- 2 tablespoons of buttermilk

- 1 garlic clove, minced

- 1/4 cup mint, chopped

- 1/2 cup of Greek yogurt, non-fat

- Salt to taste

Directions:

1. Set the Air Fryer to 390 degrees.

2. Mix all the Ingredients for the meatballs in a bowl. Roll and mold them into golf-size round pieces. Arrange in the cooking basket. Cook for 8 minutes.

3. While waiting, combine all the Ingredients for the mint yogurt in a bowl. Mix well.

4. Serve the meatballs with the mint yogurt. Top with olives and fresh mint.

5. Nutrition:

Calorie: 154

Carbohydrate: 9g

Fat: 2. 5g

Protein: 8. 6g

Fiber: 2. 4g

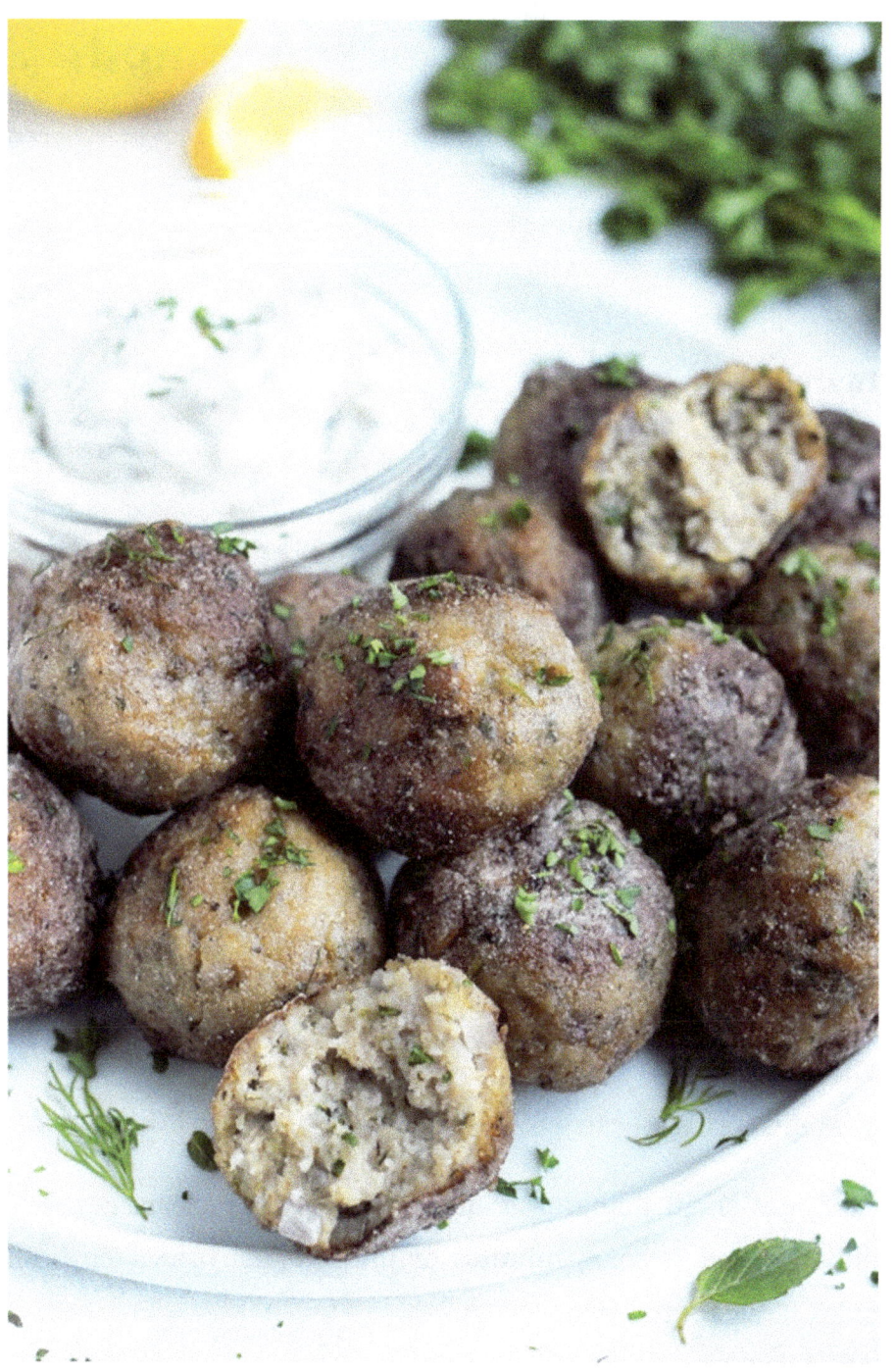

Air Fried Section And Tomato

Preparation Time: 10 minutes
Cooking Time: 5 minutes
Servings: 2

Ingredients :

- 1 aubergine, sliced thickly into 4 disks

- 1 tomato, sliced into 2 thick disks

- 2 tsp. feta cheese, reduced fat

- 2 fresh basil leaves, minced

- 2 balls, small buffalo mozzarella, reduced fat, roughly torn

- Pinch of salt

- Pinch of black pepper

Directions:

1. Preheat Air Fryer to 330 degrees F.

2. Spray small amount of oil into the Air fryer basket. Fry aubergine slices for 5 minutes or until golden brown on both sides. Transfer to a plate.

3. Fry tomato slices in batches for 5 minutes or until seared on both sides.

4. To serve, stack salad starting with an aborigine base, buffalo mozzarella, basil leaves, tomato slice, and 1/2-teaspoon feta cheese.

5. Top of with another slice of aborigine and 1/2 tsp. feta cheese. Serve.

Nutrition:
Calorie: 140.3

Carbohydrate: 26. 6

Fat: 3. 4g

Protein: 4. 2g

Fiber: 7. 3g

Cheesy Salmon Fillets

Preparation Time: 15 minutes

Cooking Time: 20 minutes

Servings: 2-3

Ingredients : For the salmon fillets

- 2 pieces, 4 oz. each salmon fillets, choose even cuts

- 1/2 cup sour cream, reduced fat

- 1/4 cup cottage cheese, reduced fat

- 1/4 cup Parmigiano-Reggiano cheese, freshly grated

Garnish:

- Spanish paprika

- 1/2 piece lemon, cut into wedges

Directions:

1. Preheat Air Fryer to 330 degrees F.

2. To make the salmon fillets, mix sour cream, cottage cheese, and Parmigiano-Reggiano cheese in a bowl.

3. Layer salmon fillets in the Air fryer basket. Fry for 20 minutes or until cheese turns golden brown.

4. To assemble, place a salmon fillet and sprinkle paprika. Garnish with lemon wedges and squeeze lemon juice on top. Serve.

Nutrition:

Calorie: 274

Carbohydrate: 1g

Fat: 19g

Protein: 24g

Fiber: 0.5g

Salmon With Asparagus

Preparation Time: 5 Minutes
Cooking Time: 10 Minutes
Servings: 3

Ingredients :

- 1 lb. Salmon, sliced into fillets

- 1 tbsp. Olive Oil

- Salt & Pepper, as needed

- 1 bunch of Asparagus, trimmed

- 2 cloves of Garlic, minced

- Zest & Juice of 1/2 Lemon

- 1 tbsp. Butter, salted

Directions:

1. Spoon in the butter and olive oil into a large pan and heat it over medium-high heat.

2. Once it becomes hot, place the salmon and season it with salt and pepper.

3. Cook for 4 minutes per side and then cook the other side.

4. Stir in the garlic and lemon zest to it.

5. Cook for further 2 minutes or until slightly browned.

6. Off the heat and squeeze the lemon juice over it.

7. Serve it hot.

Nutrition:

Calories: 409Kcal

Carbohydrates: 2. 7g

Proteins: 32. 8g

Fat: 28. 8g

Sodium: 497mg

Shrimp In Garlic Butter

Preparation Time: 5 Minutes
Cooking Time: 20 Minutes
Servings: 4

Ingredients :

- 1 lb. Shrimp, peeled & deveined

- ¼ tsp. Red Pepper Flakes

- 6 tbsp. Butter, divided

- 1/2 cup Chicken Stock

- Salt & Pepper, as needed

- 2 tbsp. Parsley, minced

- 5 cloves of Garlic, minced

- 2 tbsp. Lemon Juice

Directions:

1. Heat a large bottomed skillet over medium-high heat.

2. Spoon in two tablespoons of the butter and melt it. Add the shrimp.

3. Season it with salt and pepper. Sear for 4 minutes or until shrimp gets cooked.

4. Transfer the shrimp to a plate and stir in the garlic.

5. Sauté for 30 seconds or until aromatic.

6. Pour the chicken stock and whisk it well. Allow it to simmer for 5 to 10 minutes or until it has reduced to half.

7. Spoon the remaining butter, red pepper, and lemon juice to the sauce. Mix.

8. Continue cooking for another 2 minutes.

9. Take off the pan from the heat and add the cooked shrimp to it.

10. Garnish with parsley and transfer to the serving bowl.

11. Enjoy.

Nutrition:

Calories: 307Kcal

Carbohydrates: 3g

Proteins: 27g

Fat: 20g

Sodium: 522mg

Cobb Salad

Preparation Time: 5 Minutes

Cooking Time: 5 Minutes

Servings: 1

Ingredients :

- 4 Cherry Tomatoes, chopped

- ¼ cup Bacon, cooked & crumbled

- 1/2 of 1 Avocado, chopped

- 2 oz. Chicken Breast, shredded

- 1 Egg, hardboiled

- 2 cups Mixed Green salad

- 1 oz. Feta Cheese, crumbled

Directions:

1. Toss all the Ingredients for the Cobb salad in a large mixing bowl and toss well.

2. Serve and enjoy it.

Nutrition:

Calories: 307Kcal

Carbohydrates: 3g

Proteins: 27g

Fat: 20g

Sodium: 522mg

Seared Tuna Steak

Preparation Time: 10 Minutes
Cooking Time: 10 Minutes
Servings: 2

Ingredients :

- 1 tsp. Sesame Seeds

- 1 tbsp. Sesame Oil

- 2 tbsp. Soya Sauce

- Salt & Pepper, to taste

- 2 × 6 oz. Ahi Tuna Steaks

Directions:

1. Seasoning the tuna steaks with salt and pepper. Keep it aside on a shallow bowl.

2. In another bowl, mix soya sauce and sesame oil.

3. pour the sauce over the salmon and coat them generously with the sauce.

4. Keep it aside for 10 to 15 minutes and then heat a large skillet over medium heat.

5. Once hot, keep the tuna steaks and cook them for 3 minutes or until seared underneath.

6. Flip the fillets and cook them for a further 3 minutes.

7. Transfer the seared tuna steaks to the serving plate and slice them into 1/2 inch slices. Top with sesame seeds.

Nutrition:

Calories: 255Kcal

Fat: 9g

Carbohydrates: 1g

Proteins: 40.5g

Sodium: 293mg

Beef Chili

Preparation Time: 10 Minutes
Cooking Time: 20 Minutes
Servings: 4

Ingredients :

- 1/2 tsp. Garlic Powder

- 1 tsp. Coriander, grounded

- 1 lb. Beef, grounded

- 1/2 tsp. Sea Salt

- 1/2 tsp. Cayenne Pepper

- 1 tsp. Cumin, grounded

- 1/2 tsp. Pepper, grounded

- 1/2 cup Salsa, low-carb & no-sugar

Directions:

1. Heat a large-sized pan over medium-high heat and cook the beef in it until browned.

2. Stir in all the spices and cook them for 7 minutes or until everything is combined.

3. When the beef gets cooked, spoon in the salsa.

4. Bring the mixture to a simmer and cook for another 8 minutes or until everything comes together.

5. Take it from heat and transfer to a serving bowl.

Nutrition:

Calories: 229Kcal

Fat: 10g

Carbohydrates: 2g

Proteins: 33g

Sodium: 675mg

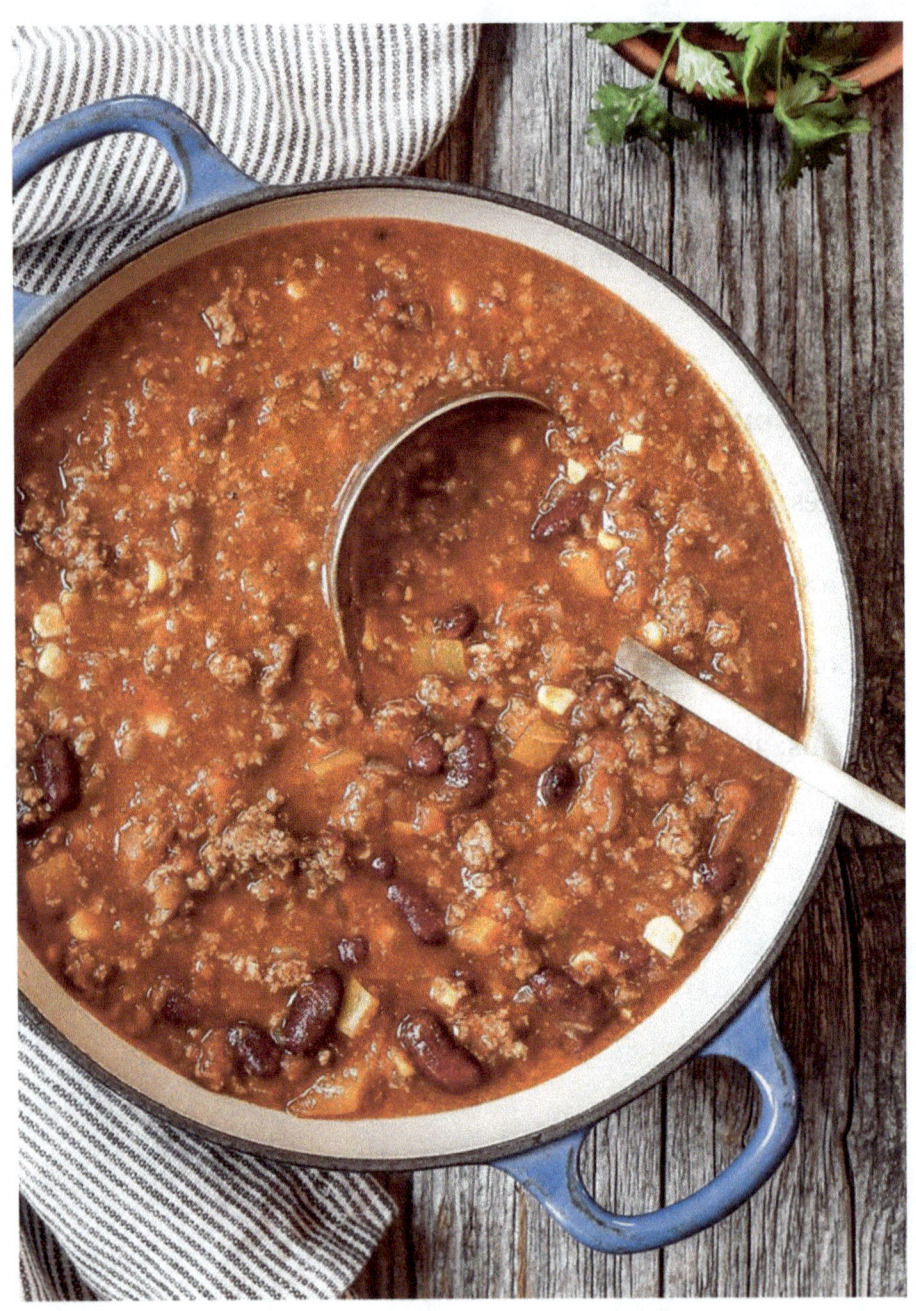

Greek Broccoli Salad

Preparation Time: 10 Minutes
Cooking Time: 15 Minutes
Servings: 4

Ingredients :

- 1 ¼ lb. Broccoli, sliced into small bites

- ¼ cup Almonds, sliced

- 1/3 cup Sun-dried Tomatoes

- ¼ cup Feta Cheese, crumbled

- ¼ cup Red Onion, sliced

For the dressing:

- 1/4 cup Olive Oil

- Dash of Red Pepper Flakes

- 1 Garlic clove, minced

- ¼ tsp. Salt

- 2 tbsp. Lemon Juice

- 1/2 tsp. Dijon Mustard

- 1 tsp. Low Carb Sweetener Syrup

- 1/2 tsp. Oregano, dried

Directions:

1. Mix broccoli, onion, almonds and sun-dried tomatoes in a large mixing bowl.

2. In another small-sized bowl, combine all the dressing Ingredients until emulsified.

3. Spoon the dressing over the broccoli salad.

4. Allow the salad to rest for 30 minutes before serving.

Nutrition:

Calories: 272Kcal

Carbohydrates: 11. 9g

Proteins: 8g

Fat: 22. 6g

Sodium: 321mg

Cheesy Cauliflower Gratin

Preparation Time: 5 Minutes
Cooking Time: 25 Minutes
Servings: 6

Ingredients :

- 6 deli slices Pepper Jack Cheese

- 4 cups Cauliflower florets

- Salt and Pepper, as needed

- 4 tbsp. Butter

- 1/3 cup Heavy Whipping Cream

Directions:

1. Mix the cauliflower, cream, butter, salt, and pepper in a safe microwave bowl and combine well.

2. Microwave the cauliflower mixture for 25 minutes on high until it becomes soft and tender.

3. Remove the Ingredients from the bowl and mash with the help of a fork.

4. Taste for seasonings and spoon in salt and pepper as required.

5. Arrange the slices of pepper jack cheese on top of the cauliflower mixture and microwave for 3 minutes until the cheese starts melting.

6. Serve warm.

Nutrition:

Calories: 421Kcal

Carbohydrates: 3g

Proteins: 19g

Fat: 37g

Sodium: 111mg

Strawberry Spinach Salad

Preparation Time: 5 Minutes
Cooking Time: 10 Minutes
Servings: 4

Ingredients :

- 4 oz. Feta Cheese, crumbled

- 8 Strawberries, sliced

- 2 oz. Almonds

- 6 Slices Bacon, thick-cut, crispy and crumbled

- 10 oz. Spinach leaves, fresh

- 2 Roma Tomatoes, diced

- 2 oz. Red Onion, sliced thinly

Directions:

1. For making this healthy salad, mix all the **Ingredients** needed to make the salad in a large-sized bowl and toss them well.

Nutrition:

Calories – 255kcal

Fat – 16g

Carbohydrates – 8g

Proteins – 14g

Sodium: 27mg

Cauliflower Mac & Cheese

Preparation Time: 5 Minutes
Cooking Time: 25 Minutes
Effort: Easy

Servings: 4

Ingredients :

- 1 Cauliflower Head, torn into florets

- Salt & Black Pepper, as needed

- ¼ cup Almond Milk, unsweetened

- ¼ cup Heavy Cream

- 3 tbsp. Butter, preferably grass-fed

- 1 cup Cheddar Cheese, shredded

Directions:

1. Preheat the oven to 450 F.

2. Melt the butter in a small microwave-safe bowl and heat it for 30 seconds.

3. Pour the melted butter over the cauliflower florets along with salt and pepper. Toss them well.

4. Place the cauliflower florets in a parchment paper-covered large baking sheet.

5. Bake them for 15 minutes or until the cauliflower is crisp-tender.

6. Once baked, mix the heavy cream, cheddar cheese, almond milk, and the remaining butter in a large microwave-safe bowl and heat it on high heat for 2 minutes or until the cheese mixture is smooth. Repeat the procedure until the cheese has melted.

7. Finally, stir in the cauliflower to the sauce mixture and coat well.

Nutrition:

Calories: 294Kcal

Fat: 23g

Carbohydrates: 7g

Proteins: 11g

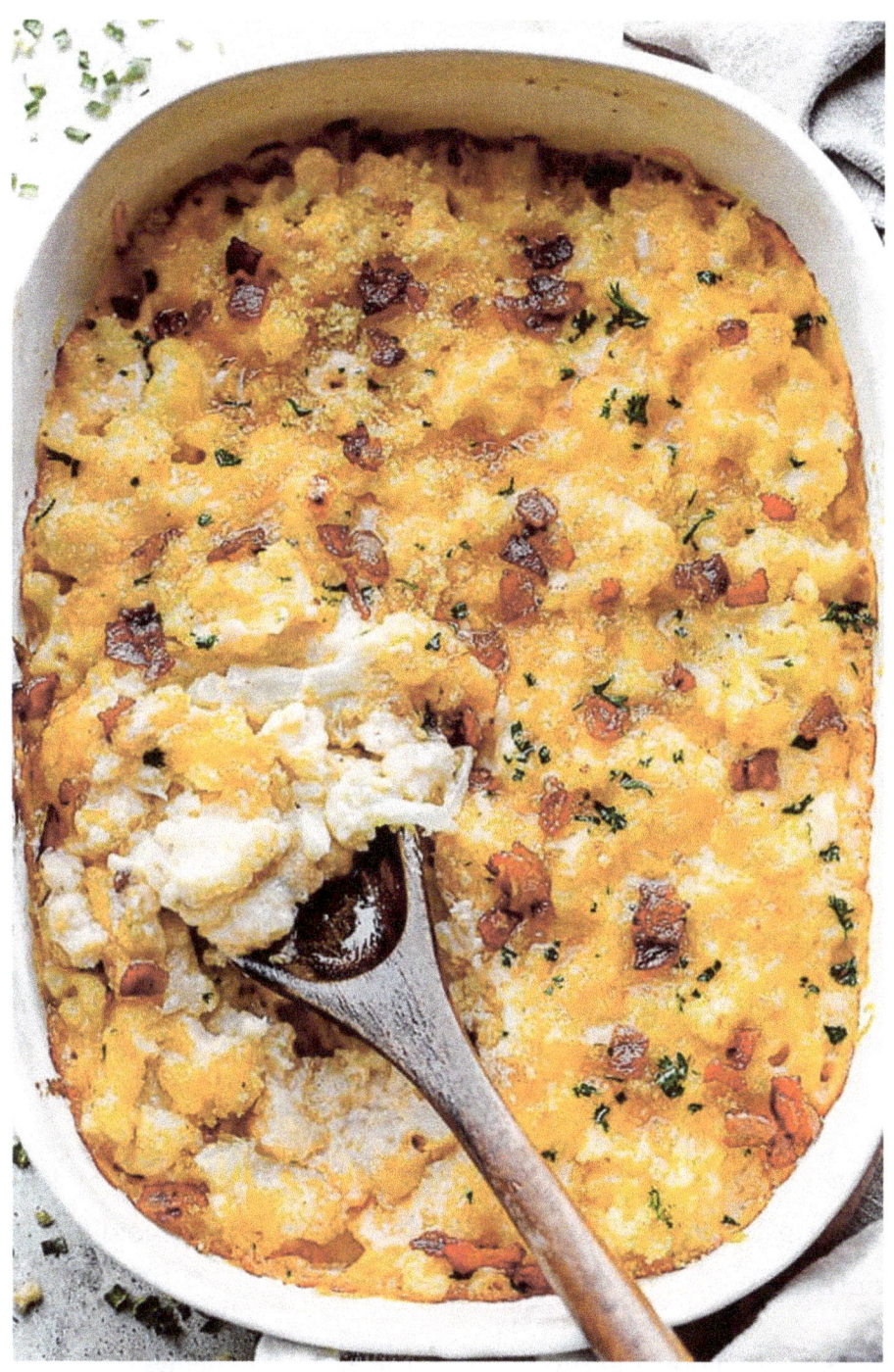

Easy Egg Salad

Preparation Time: 5 Minutes

Cooking Time: 15 to 20 Minutes

Effort: Easy

Servings: 4

Ingredients :

- 6 Eggs, preferably free-range

- ¼ tsp. Salt

- 2 tbsp. Mayonnaise

- 1 tsp. Lemon juice

- 1 tsp. Dijon mustard

- Pepper, to taste

- Lettuce leaves, to serve

Directions:

1. Keep the eggs in a saucepan of water and pour cold water until it covers the egg by another 1 inch.

2. Bring to a boil and then remove the eggs from heat.

3. Peel the eggs under cold running water.

4. Transfer the cooked eggs into a food processor and pulse them until chopped.

5. Stir in the mayonnaise, lemon juice, salt, Dijon mustard, and pepper and mix them well.

6. Taste for seasoning and add more if required.

7. Serve in the lettuce leaves.

Nutrition:

Calories – 166kcal

Fat – 14g

Carbohydrates - 0.85g

Proteins – 10g

Sodium: 132mg

Baked Chicken Legs

Preparation Time: 10 Minutes
Cooking Time: 40 Minutes
Effort: Easy

Servings: 6

Ingredients :

- 6 Chicken Legs

- ¼ tsp. Black Pepper

- ¼ cup Butter

- 1/2 tsp. Sea Salt

- 1/2 tsp. Smoked Paprika

- 1/2 tsp. Garlic Powder

Directions:

1. Preheat the oven to 425 F.

2. Pat the chicken legs with a paper towel to absorb any excess moisture.

3. Marinate the chicken pieces by first applying the butter over them and then with the seasoning. Set it aside for a few minutes.

4. Bake them for 25 minutes. Turnover and bake for further 10 minutes or until the internal temperature reaches 165 F.

5. Serve them hot.

Nutrition:

Calories – 236kL

Fat – 16g

Carbohydrates – 0g

Protein – 22g

Sodium – 314mg

Creamed Spinach

Preparation Time: 5 Minutes
Cooking Time: 10 Minutes
Effort: Easy

Servings: 4

Ingredients :

- 3 tbsp. Butter

- ¼ tsp. Black Pepper

- 4 cloves of Garlic, minced

- ¼ tsp. Sea Salt

- 10 oz. Baby Spinach, chopped

- 1 tsp. Italian Seasoning

- 1/2 cup Heavy Cream

- 3 oz. Cream Cheese

Directions:

1. Melt butter in a large sauté pan over medium heat.

2. Once the butter has melted, spoon in the garlic and sauté for 30 seconds or until aromatic.

3. Spoon in the spinach and cook for 3 to 4 minutes or until wilted.

4. Add all the remaining Ingredients to it and continuously stir until the cream cheese melts and the mixture gets thickened.

5. Serve hot

Nutrition:

Calories – 274kL

Fat – 27g

Carbohydrates – 4g

Protein – 4g

Sodium – 114mg

Stuffed Mushrooms

Preparation Time: 10 Minutes
Cooking Time: 20 Minutes
Servings: 4

Ingredients :

- 4 Portobello Mushrooms, large

- 1/2 cup Mozzarella Cheese, shredded

- 1/2 cup Marinara, low-sugar

- Olive Oil Spray

Directions:

1. Preheat the oven to 375 F.

2. Take out the dark gills from the mushrooms with the help of a spoon.

3. Keep the mushroom stem upside down and spoon it with two tablespoons of marinara sauce and mozzarella cheese.

4. Bake for 18 minutes or until the cheese is bubbly.

Nutrition:

Calories – 113kL

Fat – 6g

Carbohydrates – 4g

Protein – 7g

Sodium – 14mg

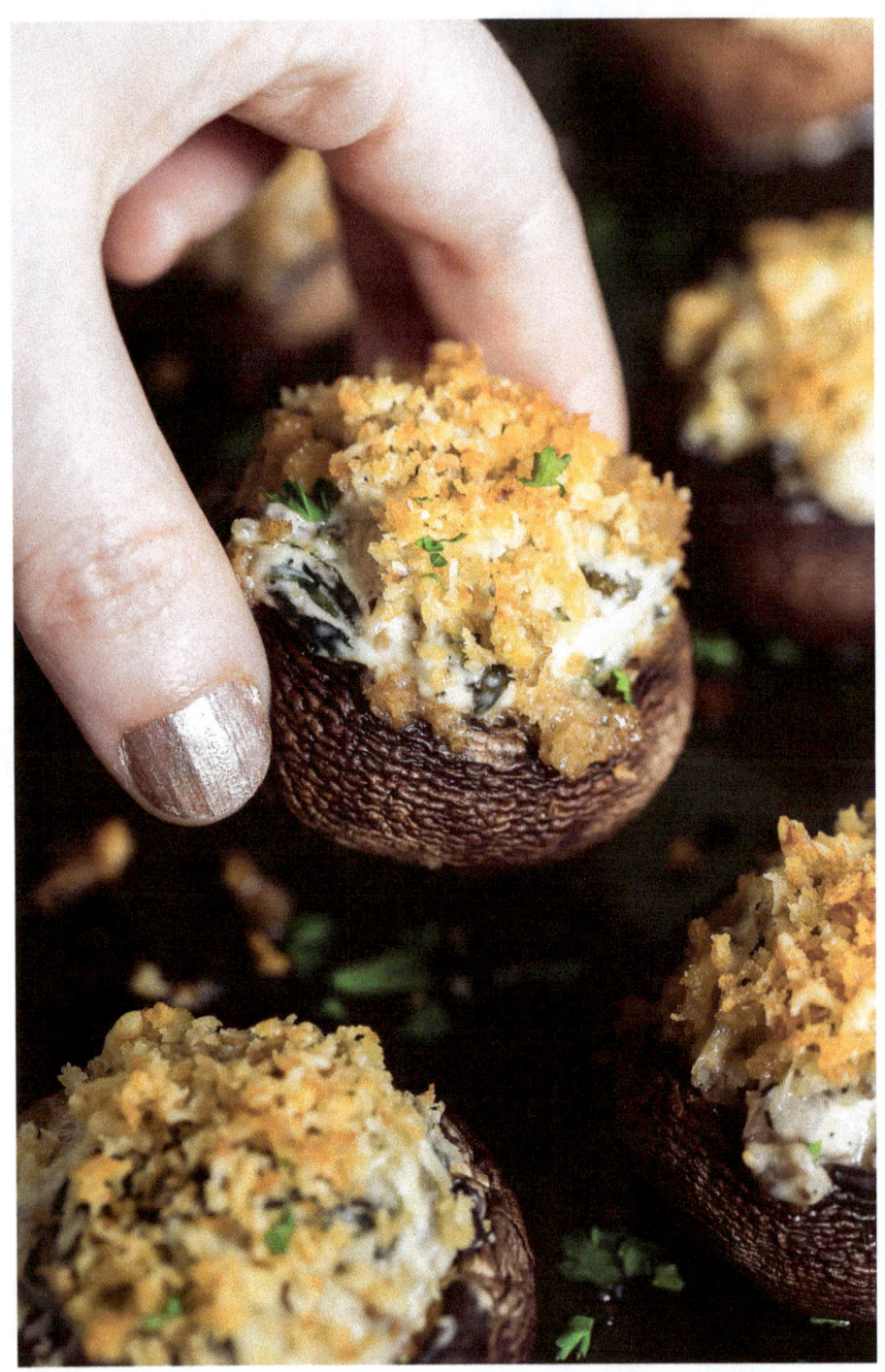

Vegetable Soup

Preparation Time: 10 Minutes
Cooking Time: 30 Minutes
Servings: 5

Ingredients :

- 8 cups Vegetable Broth

- 2 tbsp. Olive Oil

- 1 tbsp. Italian Seasoning

- 1 Onion, large & diced

- 2 Bay Leaves, dried

- 2 Bell Pepper, large & diced

- Sea Salt & Black Pepper, as needed

- 4 cloves of Garlic, minced

- 28 oz. Tomatoes, diced

- 1 Cauliflower head, medium & torn into florets

- 2 cups Green Beans, trimmed & chopped

Directions:

1. Heat oil in a Dutch oven over medium heat.

2. Once the oil becomes hot, stir in the onions and pepper.

3. Cook for 10 minutes or until the onion is softened and browned.

4. Spoon in the garlic and sauté for a minute or until fragrant.

5. Add all the remaining Ingredients to it. Mix until everything comes together.

6. Bring the mixture to a boil. Lower the heat and cook for further 20 minutes or until the vegetables have softened.

7. Serve hot.

Nutrition:

Calories – 79kL

Fat – 2g

Carbohydrates – 8g

Protein – 2g

Sodium – 187mg

Pork Chop Diane

Preparation Time: 10 minutes
Cooking Time: 20 minutes
Servings: 4

Ingredients :

- ¼ cup low-sodium chicken broth

- 1 tablespoon freshly squeezed lemon juice

- 2 teaspoons Worcestershire sauce

- 2 teaspoons Dijon mustard

- 4 (5-ounce) boneless pork top loin chops

- 1 teaspoon extra-virgin olive oil

- 1 teaspoon lemon zest

- 1 teaspoon butter

- 2 teaspoons chopped fresh chives

Directions:

1. Blend together the chicken broth, lemon juice, Worcestershire sauce, and Dijon mustard and set it aside.

2. Season the pork chops lightly.

3. Situate large skillet over medium-high heat and add the olive oil.

4. Cook the pork chops, turning once, until they are no longer pink, about 8 minutes per side.

5. Put aside the chops.

6. Pour the broth mixture into the skillet and cook until warmed through and thickened, about 2 minutes.

7. Blend lemon zest, butter, and chives.

8. Garnish with a generous spoonful of sauce.

Nutrition:
200 Calories

8g Fat

1g Carbohydrates

Autumn Pork Chops With Red Cabbage And Apples

Preparation Time: 15 minutes
Cooking Time: 30 minutes
Servings: 4

Ingredients :

- ¼ cup apple cider vinegar

- 2 tablespoons granulated sweetener

- 4 (4-ounce) pork chops, about 1 inch thick

- 1 tablespoon extra-virgin olive oil

- ½ red cabbage, finely shredded

- 1 sweet onion, thinly sliced

- 1 apple, peeled, cored, and sliced

- 1 teaspoon chopped fresh thyme

Directions:

1. Scourge together the vinegar and sweetener. Set it aside.

2. Season the pork with salt and pepper.

3. Position huge skillet over medium-high heat and add the olive oil.

4. Cook the pork chops until no longer pink, turning once, about 8 minutes per side.

5. Put chops aside.

6. Add the cabbage and onion to the skillet and sauté until the vegetables have softened, about 5 minutes.

7. Add the vinegar mixture and the apple slices to the skillet and bring the mixture to a boil.

8. Adjust heat to low and simmer, covered, for 5 additional minutes.

9. Return the pork chops to the skillet, along with any accumulated juices and thyme, cover, and cook for 5 more minutes.

Nutrition:

223 Calories

12g Carbohydrates

3g Fiber

Chipotle Chili Pork Chops

Preparation Time: 40 minutes
Cooking Time: 20 minutes
Servings: 4

Ingredients :

- Juice and zest of 1 lime

- 1 tablespoon extra-virgin olive oil

- 1 tablespoon chipotle chili powder

- 2 teaspoons minced garlic

- 1 teaspoon ground cinnamon

- Pinch sea salt

- 4 (5-ounce) pork chops

Directions:

1. Combine the lime juice and zest, oil, chipotle chili powder, garlic, cinnamon, and salt in a resealable plastic bag. Add the pork chops. Remove as much air as possible and seal the bag.

2. Marinate the chops in the refrigerator for at least 20 minutes

3. Ready the oven to 400°F and set a rack on a baking sheet. Let the chops rest at room temperature for 15 minutes, then arrange them on the rack and discard the remaining marinade.

4. Roast the chops until cooked through, turning once, about 10 minutes per side.

5. Serve with lime wedges.

Nutrition:

204 Calories

1g Carbohydrates

1g Sugar

Orange-Marinated Pork Tenderloin

Preparation Time: 20 minutes
Cooking Time: 30 minutes
Servings: 4

Ingredients :

- ¼ cup freshly squeezed orange juice

- 2 teaspoons orange zest

- 2 teaspoons minced garlic

- 1 teaspoon low-sodium soy sauce

- 1 teaspoon grated fresh ginger

- 1 teaspoon honey

- 1½ pounds pork tenderloin roast

- 1 tablespoon extra-virgin olive oil

Directions:

1. Blend together the orange juice, zest, garlic, soy sauce, ginger, and honey.

2. Pour the marinade into a resealable plastic bag and add the pork tenderloin.

3. Remove as much air as possible and seal the bag. Marinate the pork in the refrigerator, turning the bag a few times, for 20 minutes.

4. Preheat the oven to 400°F.

5. Pull out tenderloin from the marinade and discard the marinade.

6. Position big ovenproof skillet over medium-high heat and add the oil.

7. Sear the pork tenderloin on all sides, about 5 minutes in total.

8. Position skillet to the oven and roast for 25 minutes.

9. Put aside for 10 minutes before serving.

Nutrition:

228 Calories

4g Carbohydrates

3g Sugar

Homestyle Herb Meatballs

Preparation Time: 10 minutes
Cooking Time: 15 minutes
Servings: 4

Ingredients :

- ½ pound lean ground pork

- ½ pound lean ground beef

- 1 sweet onion, finely chopped

- ¼ cup bread crumbs

- 2 tablespoons chopped fresh basil

- 2 teaspoons minced garlic

- 1 egg

Directions:

1. Preheat the oven to 350°F.

2. Ready baking tray with parchment paper and set it aside.

3. In a large bowl, mix together the pork, beef, onion, bread crumbs, basil, garlic, egg, salt, and pepper until very well mixed.

4. Roll the meat mixture into 2-inch meatballs.

5. Transfer the meatballs to the baking sheet and bake until they are browned and cooked through, about 15 minutes.

6. Serve the meatballs with your favorite marinara sauce and some steamed green beans.

Nutrition:

332 Calories

13g Carbohydrates

3g Sugar

Lime-Parsley Lamb Cutlets

Preparation Time: 40 minutes
Cooking Time: 10 minutes
Servings: 4

Ingredients :

- ¼ cup extra-virgin olive oil

- ¼ cup freshly squeezed lime juice

- 2 tablespoons lime zest

- 2 tablespoons chopped fresh parsley

- 12 lamb cutlets (about 1½ pounds total)

Directions:

1. Scourge the oil, lime juice, zest, parsley, salt, and pepper.

2. Pour marinade to a resealable plastic bag.

3. Add the cutlets to the bag and remove as much air as possible before sealing.

4. Marinate the lamb in the refrigerator for about 40 minutes, turning the bag several times.

5. Preheat the oven to broil.

6. Remove the chops from the bag and arrange them on an aluminum foil–lined baking sheet. Discard the marinade.

7. Broil the chops for 4 minutes per side for medium doneness.

8. Let the chops rest for 5 minutes before serving.

Nutrition:

413 Calories

1g Carbohydrates

31g Protein

Mediterranean Steak Sandwiches

Preparation Time: 10 minutes

Cooking Time: 10 minutes

Servings: 4

Ingredients :

- 2 tablespoons extra-virgin olive oil

- 2 tablespoons balsamic vinegar

- 2 teaspoons garlic

- 2 teaspoons lemon juice

- 2 teaspoons fresh oregano

- 1 teaspoon fresh parsley

- 1-pound flank steak

- 4 whole-wheat pitas

- 2 cups shredded lettuce

- 1 red onion, thinly sliced

- 1 tomato, chopped

- 1 ounce low-sodium feta cheese

Directions:

1. Scourge olive oil, balsamic vinegar, garlic, lemon juice, oregano, and parsley.

2. Add the steak to the bowl, turning to coat it completely.

3. Marinate the steak for 30 minutes in the refrigerator, turning it over several times.

4. Preheat the broiler. Line a baking sheet with aluminum foil.

5. Put steak out of the bowl and discard the marinade.

6. Situate steak on the baking sheet and broil for 5 minutes per side for medium.

7. Set aside for 10 minutes before slicing.

8. Stuff the pitas with the sliced steak, lettuce, onion, tomato, and feta.

Nutrition:

344 Calories

22g Carbohydrates

3g Fiber

Roasted Beef With Peppercorn Sauce

Preparation Time: 10 minutes
Cooking Time: 90 minutes
Servings: 4

Ingredients :

- 1½ pounds top rump beef roast

- 3 teaspoons extra-virgin olive oil

- 3 shallots, minced

- 2 teaspoons minced garlic

- 1 tablespoon green peppercorns

- 2 tablespoons dry sherry

- 2 tablespoons all-purpose flour

- 1 cup sodium-free beef broth

Directions:

1. Heat the oven to 300°F.

2. Season the roast with salt and pepper.

3. Position huge skillet over medium-high heat and add 2 teaspoons of olive oil.

4. Brown the beef on all sides, about 10 minutes in total, and transfer the roast to a baking dish.

5. Roast until desired doneness, about 40 minutes for medium. When the roast has been in the oven for 30 minutes, start the sauce.

6. In a medium saucepan over medium-high heat, sauté the shallots in the remaining 1 teaspoon of olive oil until translucent, about 4 minutes.

7. Stir in the garlic and peppercorns, and cook for another minute. Whisk in the sherry to deglaze the pan.

8. Whisk in the flour to form a thick paste, cooking for 1 minute and stirring constantly.

9. Fill in the beef broth and whisk for 4 minutes. Season the sauce.

10. Serve the beef with a generous spoonful of sauce.

Nutrition:

330 Calories

4g Carbohydrates

36g Protein

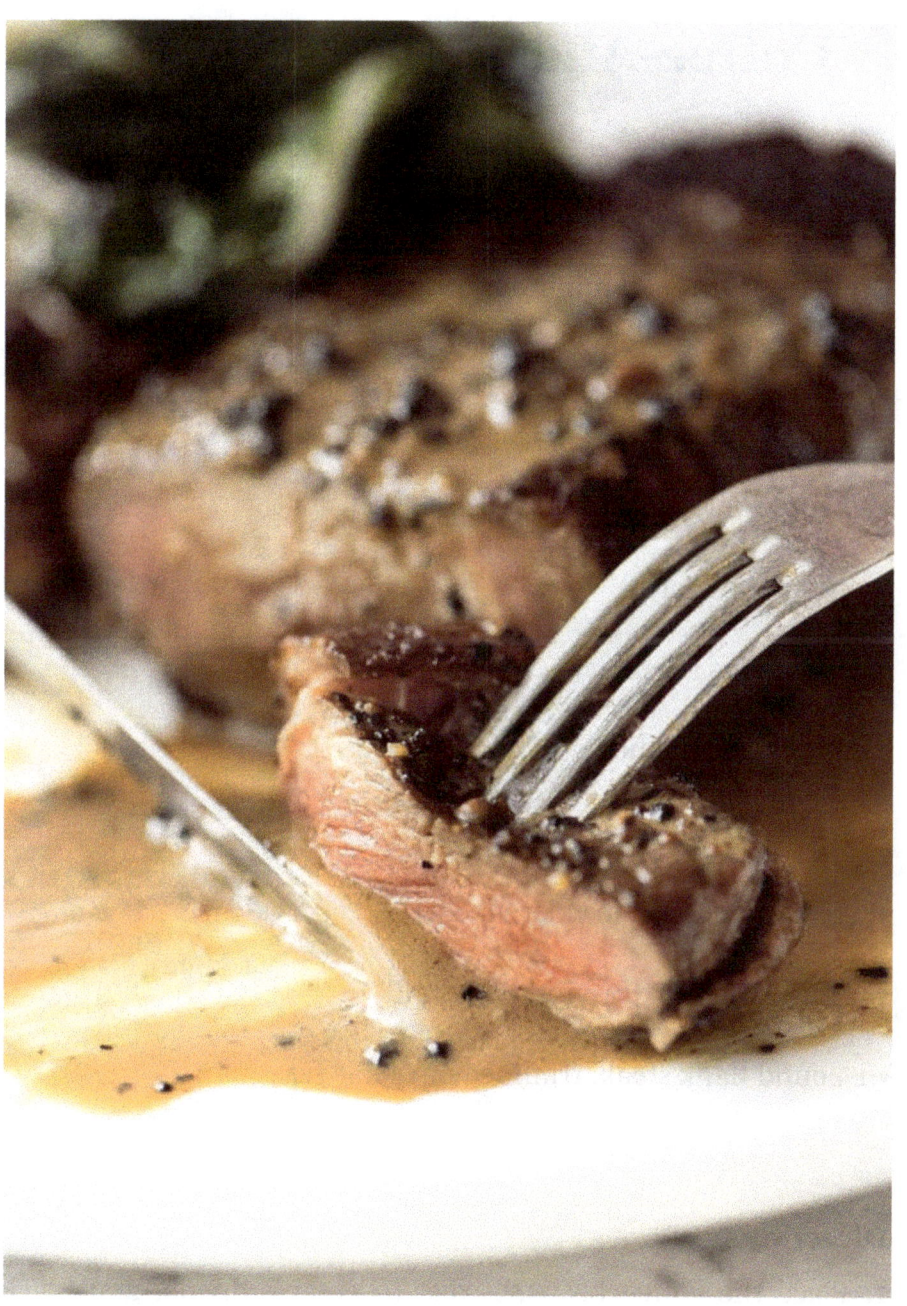

Coffee-And-Herb-Marinated Steak

Preparation Time: 20 minutes
Cooking Time: 10 minutes
Servings: 3

Ingredients :

- ¼ cup whole coffee beans

- 2 teaspoons garlic

- 2 teaspoons rosemary

- 2 teaspoons thyme

- 1 teaspoon black pepper

- 2 tablespoons apple cider vinegar

- 2 tablespoons extra-virgin olive oil

- 1-pound flank steak, trimmed of visible fat

Directions:

1. Place the coffee beans, garlic, rosemary, thyme, and black pepper in a coffee grinder or food processor and pulse until coarsely ground.

2. Transfer the coffee mixture to a resealable plastic bag and add the vinegar and oil. Shake to combine.

3. Add the flank steak and squeeze the excess air out of the bag. Seal it. Marinate the steak in the refrigerator for at least 20 minutes, occasionally turning the bag over.

4. Preheat the broiler. Line a baking sheet with aluminum foil.

5. Pull the steak out and discard the marinade.

6. Position steak on the baking sheet and broil until it is done to your liking.

7. Put aside for 10 minutes before cutting it.

8. Serve with your favorite side dish.

Nutrition:

313 Calories

20g Fat

31g Protein

Traditional Beef Stroganoff

Preparation Time: 10 minutes
Cooking Time: 30 minutes
Servings: 4

Ingredients :

- 1 teaspoon extra-virgin olive oil

- 1-pound top sirloin, cut into thin strips

- 1 cup sliced button mushrooms

- ½ sweet onion, finely chopped

- 1 teaspoon minced garlic

- 1 tablespoon whole-wheat flour

- ½ cup low-sodium beef broth

- ¼ cup dry sherry

- ½ cup fat-free sour cream

- 1 tablespoon chopped fresh parsley

Directions:

1. Position the skillet over medium-high heat and add the oil.

2. Sauté the beef until browned, about 10 minutes, then remove the beef with a slotted spoon to a plate and set it aside.

3. Add the mushrooms, onion, and garlic to the skillet and sauté until lightly browned, about 5 minutes.

4. Whisk in the flour and then whisk in the beef broth and sherry.

5. Return the sirloin to the skillet and bring the mixture to a boil.

6. Reduce the heat to low and simmer until the beef is tender, about 10 minutes.

7. Stir in the sour cream and parsley. Season with salt and pepper.

Nutrition:

257 Calories

6g Carbohydrates

1g Fiber

Chicken And Roasted Vegetable Wraps

Preparation Time: 10 minutes

Cooking Time: 20 minutes

Servings: 4

Ingredients :

- ½ small eggplant

- 1 red bell pepper

- 1 medium zucchini

- ½ small red onion, sliced

- 1 tablespoon extra-virgin olive oil

- 2 (8-ounce) cooked chicken breasts, sliced

- 4 whole-wheat tortilla wraps

Directions:

1. Preheat the oven to 400°F.

2. Wrap baking sheet with foil and set it aside.

3. In a large bowl, toss the eggplant, bell pepper, zucchini, and red onion with the olive oil.

4. Transfer the vegetables to the baking sheet and lightly season with salt and pepper.

5. Roast the vegetables until soft and slightly charred, about 20 minutes.

6. Divide the vegetables and chicken into four portions.

7. Wrap 1 tortilla around each portion of chicken and grilled vegetables, and serve.

Nutrition:
483 Calories

45g Carbohydrates

3g Fiber

Spicy Chicken Cacciatore

Preparation Time: 20 minutes
Cooking Time: 25 minutes
Servings: 6

Ingredients :

- 1 (2-pound) chicken

- ¼ cup all-purpose flour

- 2 tablespoons extra-virgin olive oil

- 3 slices bacon

- 1 sweet onion

- 2 tespoons minced garlic

- 4 ounces button mushrooms, halved

- 1 (28-ounce) can low-sodium stewed tomatoes

- ½ cup red wine

- 2 teaspoons chopped fresh oregano

Directions:

1. Cut the chicken into pieces: 2 drumsticks, 2 thighs, 2 wings, and 4 breast pieces.

2. Dredge the chicken pieces in the flour and season each piece with salt and pepper.

3. Place a large skillet over medium-high heat and add the olive oil.

4. Brown the chicken pieces on all sides, about 20 minutes in total. Transfer the chicken to a plate.

5. Cook chopped bacon to the skillet for 5 minutes. With a slotted spoon, transfer the cooked bacon to the same plate as the chicken.

6. Pour off most of the oil from the skillet, leaving just a light coating. Sauté the onion, garlic, and mushrooms in the skillet until tender, about 4 minutes.

7. Stir in the tomatoes, wine, oregano, and red pepper flakes.

8. Bring the sauce to a boil. Return the chicken and bacon, plus any accumulated juices from the plate, to the skillet.

9. Reduce the heat to low and simmer until the chicken is tender, about 30 minutes.

Nutrition:

230 Calories

14g Carbohydrates

2g Fiber

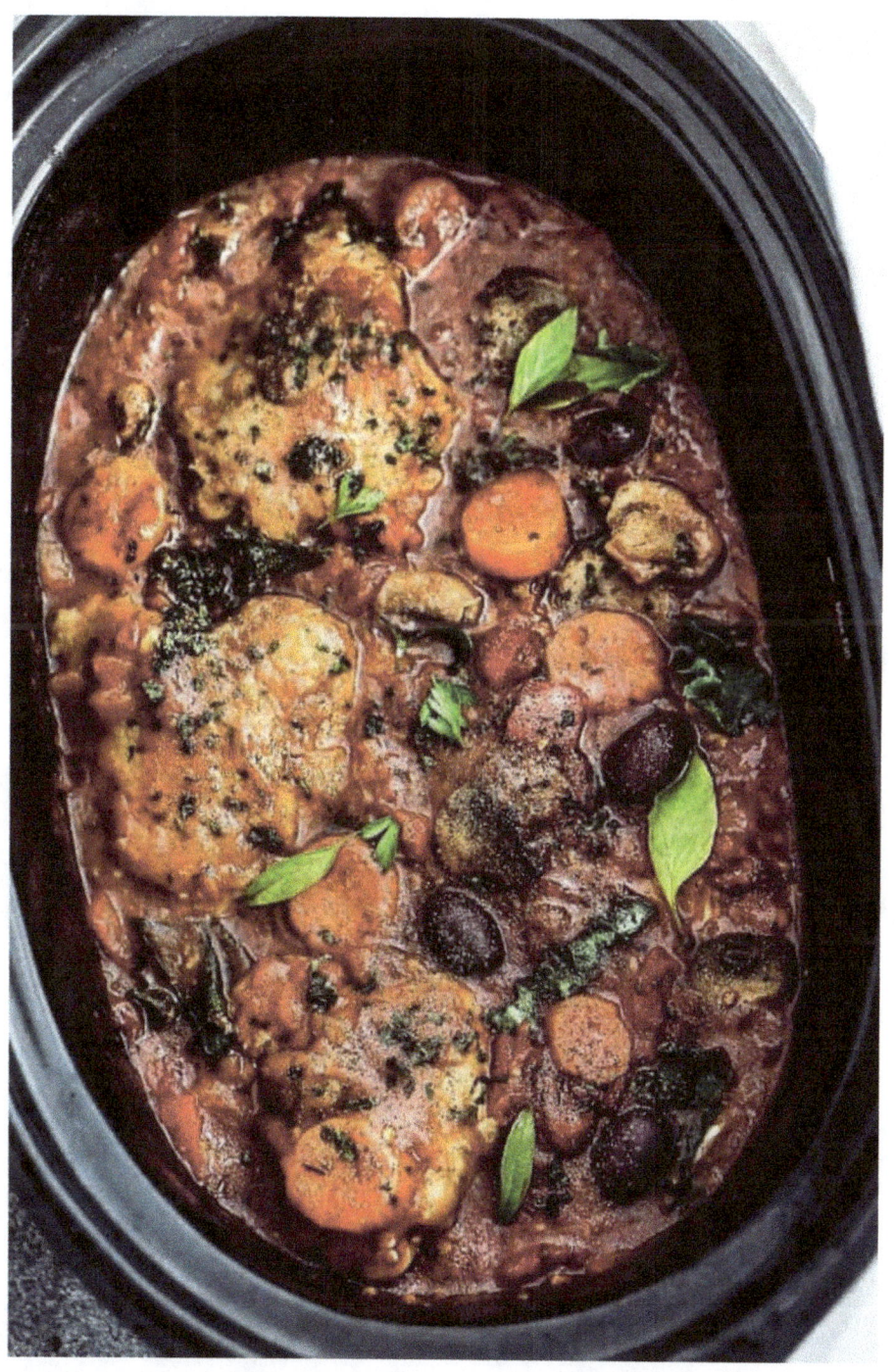

www.ingramcontent.com/pod-product-compliance
Lightning Source LLC
Chambersburg PA
CBHW070725030426
42336CB00013B/1918